Lean & Green Air Fryer Cookbook for Beginners

The Perfect Cookbook for Tasty and Easy Recipes

Roxana Sutton

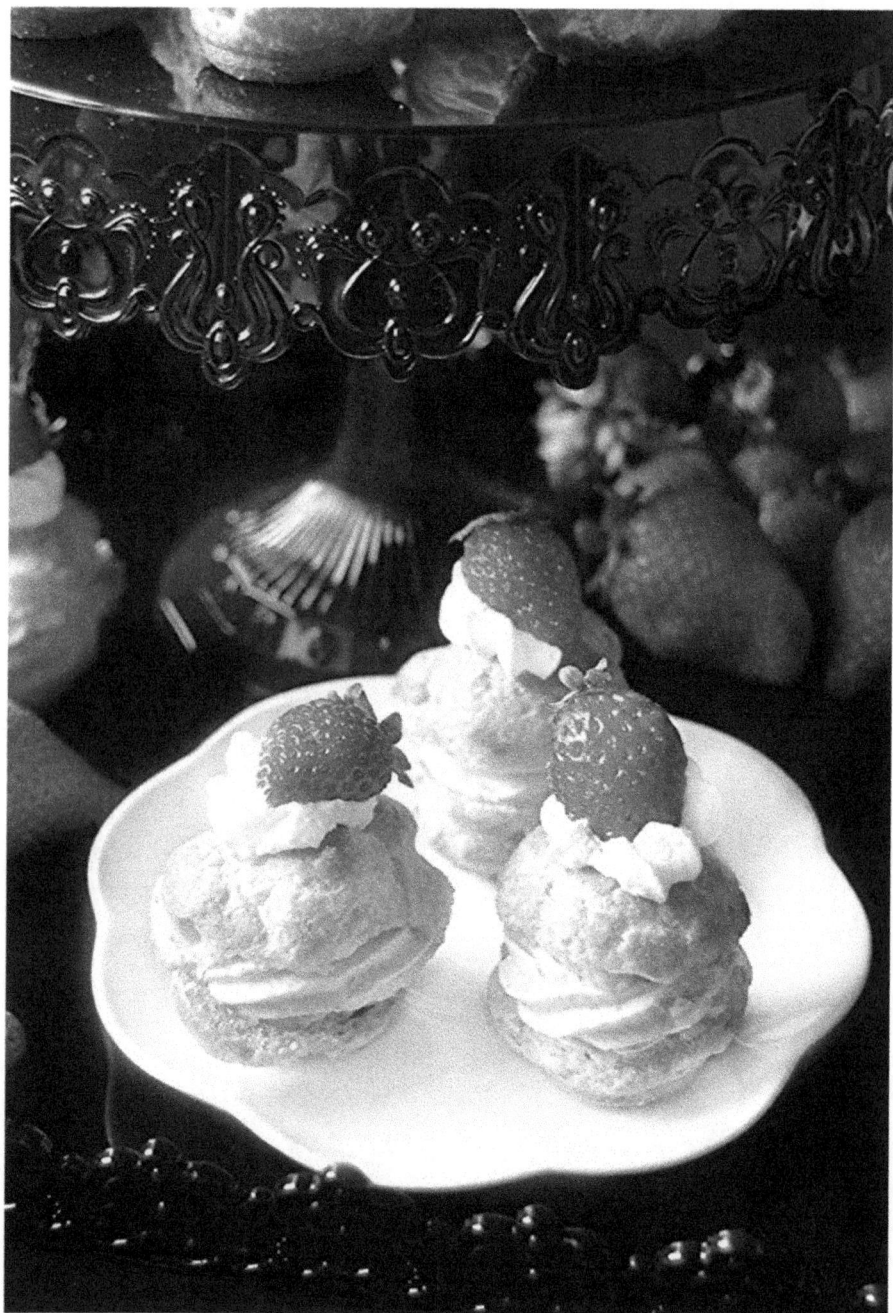

Sesame Crusted Sweet Potato Cakes

Prep Time: 15 mins

Cook Time: 10 mins

Ingredients

- 400 g mashed sweet potato
- 70 g tapioca starch
- 20 g cake flour sugar to taste
- 1/4 cup toasted sesame seeds

Instructions

In a large mixing bowl, combine the mashed sweet potato, tapioca starch, cake flour, and sugar until homogenous.

Roll the dough into a long strip. Cut the dough into one-inch pieces and roll them into a round ball. Flatten the balls with the palm of your hand to form patties.

Sprinkle sesame seeds onto the patties and press the sesame seeds into the patties. Repeat this step for the other side.

Spray oil to both sides and air fry at 380F (190C) for about 10 minutes, flip once in between.

Nutrition

Calories: 108kcal | Carbohydrates: 21g | Protein: 2g | Fat: 2g | Saturated Fat: 1g | Sodium: 28mg | Potassium: 190mg | Fiber: 2g | Sugar: 2g | Vitamin C: 1mg | Calcium: 61mg | Iron: 1mg

Strawberry Puff Pastry Twists

Prep Time: 10 mins

Cook Time: 10 mins

Ingredients

- 1 Puff pastry sheet defrosted and cut into two equal pieces
- 4-5 Tablespoon strawberry preserve

Instructions

Spread the strawberry preserve on one piece of the puff pastry. Place the other piece on top. Using a sharp knife or a dough blade, cut the pastry dough "sandwich" into 1/2 inch wide strips.

Twist each strip and place them in a parchment paper-lined fryer basket and air fry at 360F (180C) for 9-10 minutes, flip once in between.

Let cool completely before serving.

Nutrition

Calories: 393kcal | Carbohydrates: 41g | Protein: 5g | Fat: 23g | Saturated Fat: 6g | Sodium: 159mg | Potassium: 53mg | Fiber: 1g | Sugar: 10g | Vitamin C: 2mg | Calcium: 10mg | Iron: 2mg

Maple Sponge Cake

Prep Time: 10 mins

Cook Time: 15 mins

Ingredients

- 50 g cake flour
- 1/2 teaspoon baking powder
- 35 g melted butter and let it cool to almost room temperature
- 2 tablespoon milk
- 2 1/2 tablespoon maple syrup
- 1/4 teaspoon vanilla extract
- 3 large eggs

Instructions

Crack 3 eggs and put the egg whites in the mixing bowl and egg yolks in a medium-sized bowl.

To the egg yolks, add in the cooled butter, maple syrup, and vanilla extract and mix until well combined.

In a separate large bowl, sieve the cake flour and baking powder and mix them. Pour the egg yolk mixture into this large bowl and gently whisk to combine the wet and dry ingredients to form a thick batter.

In the meantime, use the electric mixer (or a whisk) to beat the egg whites until they can form a stiff peak. When done, pour this fluffy egg whites into the batter and gently combine them with a spatula until it is almost homogenous.

Put the muffin tins inside the fryer basket, hold them down with a steamer rack and preheat the air fryer at 400F (200C) for about 2 minutes.

Pour the batter into the preheated muffin tins and air fry at 260F (130C) for about 13 minutes until the toothpick comes out clean. Air fry at 380F (190C) again for about 1-2 minutes until the color turns golden brown.

Nutrition

Calories: 195kcal | Carbohydrates: 18g | Protein: 6g | Fat: 11g | Saturated Fat: 6g | Cholesterol: 142mg | Sodium: 114mg | Potassium: 147mg | Fiber: 1g | Sugar: 8g | Calcium: 62mg | Iron: 1mg

Almond Flour Chocolate Banana Nut Brownie

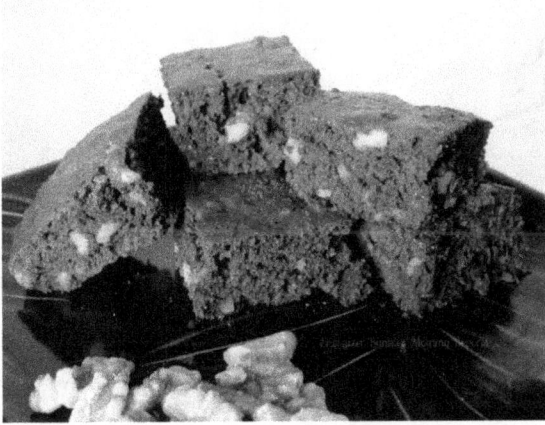

Prep Time: 5 mins

Cook Time: 8 mins

Ingredients For Brownie:

- 1 large ripe banana
- 3 Tablespoons coconut oil melted
- 1 teaspoon vanilla extract
- 1 1/2 cups almond flour
- 1/3 cup chocolate whey protein powder
- 1/2 teaspoon baking soda
- 1/4 teaspoon salt

Other Ingredients:

- 1/4 cup chocolate chips or to taste
- 1/4 cup chopped walnuts or to taste

Instructions

In a mixing bowl, mix all the ingredients, except chocolate chips and walnuts, until well combined. Fold in the chocolate chips and walnuts if desired.

Line parchment paper in a 7-inch springform pan. Pour the batter into the pan and air fry at 300F (150C) for about 8 minutes.

Let cool on a cooling rack. When cooled, cut it into 1-inch squares to serve.

Nutrition

Calories:307kcal | Carbohydrates: 16g | Protein: 7g | Fat: 26g | Saturated Fat: 8g | Cholesterol: 1mg | Sodium: 194mg | Potassium: 92mg | Fiber: 4g | Sugar: 8g | Vitamin C: 2mg | Calcium: 72mg | Iron: 1mg

Marshmallow Chocolate Chip Explosion Cookies

Prep Time: 10 mins

Cook Time: 10 mins

Ingredients

- 2/3 cup all-purpose flour
- 1/4 teaspoon baking soda
- 1/4 cup unsalted butter softened at room temperature
- 1/3 cup brown sugar
- 1 egg yolk
- 1/2 teaspoon vanilla extract
- 1/2 cup chocolate chips or to taste
- 1/4 cup marshmallow or to taste chopped into about 1/4 inch cubes
- 1/8 teaspoon salt

Instructions

Preheat the air fryer at 350F (175C) for about 3-4 minutes.

Line a small cookie sheet or bakeware with parchment paper and set it aside. This step is crucial. Without some kind of bakeware under the parchment paper, the edges of the paper may be lifted off during the air frying process which may cause the cookies to bunch together.

In a medium bowl, combine the flour, baking soda, and salt.

In a large bowl, whisk together the butter and brown sugar until smooth. Add in the egg yolk and vanilla extract and whisk again.

Combine the two bowls and mix well. Scoop one tablespoonful of the dough and roll it into a ball. Flatten it with the palm of your hand and put the desired amount of marshmallow and chocolate chip in the middle. Wrap the dough around to form a ball again. Place the balls of dough on the parchment paper, making sure they are about 2 inches apart from each other.

Air fry at 350F (175C) for 5-6 minutes until the cookies look crispy. Remove the cookies and let them cool on a rack. Repeat the same process for the remaining dough if necessary.

For your enjoyment, my little baker recommends the cookies to be warmed up a bit and topped with a scoop of ice cream.

Nutrition

Calories: 257kcal | Carbohydrates: 35g | Protein: 3g | Fat: 12g | Saturated Fat: 7g | Cholesterol: 55mg | Sodium: 112mg | Potassium: 31mg | Fiber: 1g | Sugar: 23g | Calcium: 36mg | Iron: 1mg

Coffee Cake

Prep Time: 15 mins

Cook Time: 30 mins

Ingredients

- 1/2 cup oil
- 1 egg beaten
- 1/2 teaspoon vanilla extract
- 1/2 cup milk
- 1/2 cup sugar
- 1 1/2 cup cake flour
- 1 1/2 teaspoon baking powder
- 1/4 teaspoon salt
- 1/2 cup brown sugar
- 1 teaspoon cinnamon
- 1/4 cup melted butter

Instructions

In a medium bowl, prepare streusel by combining brown sugar and cinnamon. Divide the streusel into two equal portions.

In a large mixing bowl, combine oil, eggs, vanilla, and milk. In a medium bowl, blend sugar, flour, baking powder, and salt. Then, combine egg mixture with flour mixture, mix well, then divide the batter into two equal parts.

Lightly grease the loaf pans. Pour 1/2 of the batter into each pan. Sprinkle 1/2 of streusel into the pan and top it off with the remaining batter

Sprinkle the remaining streusel on top and drizzle with melted butter.

Air fry at 320F (160C) for about 30 minutes until the toothpick comes out clean.

Nutrition

Calories: 379kcal | Carbohydrates: 44g | Protein: 4g | Fat: 21g | Saturated Fat: 5g | Cholesterol: 37mg | Sodium: 143mg | Potassium: 145mg | Fiber: 1g | Sugar: 27g | Calcium: 72mg | Iron: 1mg

Apple French Toast Cups

Prep Time: 10 mins

Cook Time: 15 mins

Ingredients

- 1 apple peeled and cubed
- 1 Tablespoon butter
- 6 oz bread or bread ends cut into one-inch cubes
- 1/3 cup brown sugar
- 1 teaspoons cornstarch
- 3 eggs
- 2/3 cups milk
- 1/2 teaspoon vanilla extract
- 1/2 teaspoon cinnamon
- 1 Tablespoon maple syrup

Instructions

In a microwave-safe bowl, microwave the apple cubes with butter for about 3 minutes until the apples are tender. Let cool for a few minutes.

Combine the bread, sugar, and cornstarch in a large mixing bowl.

In a separate bowl, mix the eggs, milk, vanilla, cinnamon, apple (and its juices) and maple syrup then pour this mixture into the bread bowl and gently combine all ingredients.

Scoop the mixture into a lightly greased muffin tin and air fry at 320F (160C) for about 12-14 minutes until the surface is golden brown.

Nutrition

Calories:336kcal | Carbohydrates: 55g | Protein: 10g | Fat: 9g | Saturated Fat: 4g | Cholesterol: 134mg | Sodium: 292mg | Potassium: 272mg | Fiber: 3g | Sugar: 33g | Vitamin C: 2mg | Calcium: 152mg | Iron: 2mg

Air Fryer Apple Pies

Prep Time:30 mins

Cook Time: 15 mins

Total Time: 45 mins

Ingredient

- 4 tablespoons butter
- 6 tablespoons brown sugar
- 1 teaspoon ground cinnamon
- 2 medium granny smith apples, diced
- 1 teaspoon cornstarch
- 2 teaspoons cold water
- ½ (14 ounces) package pastry for a 9-inch double-crust pie
- Cooking spray
- ½ tablespoon grapeseed oil
- ¼ cup powdered sugar
- 1 teaspoon milk, or more as needed

Instructions

Combine apples, butter, brown sugar, and cinnamon in a non-stick skillet. Cook over medium heat until apples have softened, about 5 minutes.

Dissolve cornstarch in cold water. Stir into apple mixture and cook until sauce thickens about 1 minute. Remove apple pie filling from heat and set aside to cool while you prepare the crust.

Unroll pie crust on a lightly floured surface and roll out slightly to smooth the surface of the dough. Cut the dough into rectangles small enough so that 2 can fit in your air fryer at one time. Repeat with the remaining crust until you have 8 eɒual rectangles, re-rolling some of the scraps of dough if needed. Wet the outer edges of 4 rectangles with water and place some apple filling in the center about 1/2-inch from the edges. Roll out the remaining 4 rectangles so that they are slightly larger than the filled ones. Place these rectangles on top of the filling; crimp the edges with a fork to seal. Cut 4 small slits in the tops of the pies.

Spray the basket of an air fryer with cooking spray. Brush the tops of 2 pies with grapeseed oil and transfer pies to the air fryer basket using a spatula.

Insert basket and set the temperature to 385 degrees F (195 degrees C). Bake until golden brown, about 8 minutes. Remove pies from the basket and repeat with the remaining 2 pies.

Mix powdered sugar and milk in a small bowl. Brush glaze on warm pies and allow to dry. Serve pies warm or at room temperature.

Nutrition Facts

Calories: 497| Protein: 3.2g| Carbohydrates: 59.7g| Fat: 28.6g| Cholesterol: 30.5mg| Sodium: 327.6mg.

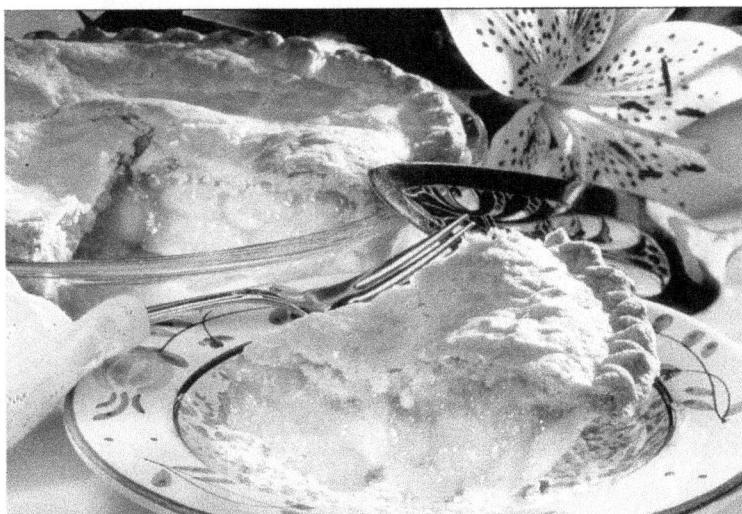

Air Fryer Oreos

Prep Time: 5 mins

Cook Time: 5 mins

Total Time: 10 mins

Ingredient

- ½ Cup complete pancake mix
- ⅓ cup water Cooking spray
- 9 chocolate sandwich cookies (such as oreo®)
- 1 tablespoon confectioners' sugar, or to taste

Instructions

Mix pancake mix and water until well combined.

Line an air fryer basket with parchment paper. Spray parchment paper with nonstick cooking spray. Dip each cookie into the pancake mixture and place it in the basket. Make sure they are not touching; cook in batches if necessary.

Preheat the air fryer to 400 degrees F (200 degrees C). Add basket and cook for 4 to 5 minutes; flip and cook until golden brown, 2 to 3 minutes more. Sprinkle with confectioners' sugar.

Nutrition Facts

Calories: 77| Protein: 1.2g| Carbohydrates: 13.7g| Fat: 2.1g| Sodium: 156mg.

Air Fryer Churros

Prep Time: 5 mins

Cook Time: 15 mins

Additional Time: 5 mins

Total Time: 25 mins

Ingredient

- ¼ cup butter
- ½ cup milk 1 pinch salt
- ½ cup all-purpose flour
- 2 eggs
- ¼ cup white sugar
- ½ teaspoon ground cinnamon

Instructions

Melt butter in a saucepan over medium-high heat. Pour in milk and add salt. Lower heat to medium and bring to a boil, continuously stirring with a wooden spoon. Quickly add flour all at once. Keep stirring until the dough comes together.

Remove from heat and let cool for 5 to 7 minutes. Mix in eggs with the wooden spoon until the pastry comes together. Spoon dough into a pastry bag fitted with a large star tip. Pipe dough into strips straight into the air fryer basket.

Air fry churros at 340 degrees F (175 degrees C) for 5 minutes.

Meanwhile, combine sugar and cinnamon in a small bowl and pour onto a shallow plate. Remove fried churros from the air fryer and roll in the cinnamon-sugar mixture.

Nutrition Facts

Calories: 173| Protein: 3.9g| Carbohydrates: 17.5g| Fat: 9.8g| Cholesterol: 84mg| Sodium: 112.2mg.

Air Fryer Apple Fritters

Prep Time: 15 mins

Cook Time: 10 mins

Total Time: 25 mins

Ingredient

- Cooking spray
- 1 cup all-purpose flour
- ¼ cup white sugar
- ¼ cup milk
- 1 egg
- 1 ½ teaspoons baking powder
- 1 pinch salt
- 2 tablespoons white sugar
- ½ teaspoon ground cinnamon
- 1 apple - peeled, cored, and chopped

Glaze:

- ½ cup confectioners' sugar
- 1 tablespoon milk
- ½ teaspoon caramel extract
- ¼ teaspoon ground cinnamon

Instructions

Preheat an air fryer to 350 degrees F (175 degrees C). Place a parchment paper round into the bottom of the air fryer. Spray with nonstick cooking spray.

Mix flour, 1/4 cup sugar, milk, egg, baking powder, and salt together in a small bowl. Stir until combined.

Mix 2 tablespoons sugar with cinnamon in another bowl and sprinkle over apples until coated. Mix apples into the flour mixture until combined.

Drop fritters using a cookie scoop onto the bottom of the air fryer basket.

Air-fry in the preheated fryer for 5 minutes. Flip fritters and cook until golden, about 5 minutes more. Meanwhile, mix confectioners' sugar, milk, caramel extract, and cinnamon in a bowl. Transfer fritters to a cooling rack and drizzle with glaze.

Nutrition Facts

Calories: 297| Protein: 5.5g| Carbohydrates: 64.9g| Fat: 2.1g| Cholesterol: 48mg| Sodium: 248.6mg.

Air Fryer Roasted Bananas

Prep Time: 2 mins

Cook Time: 7 mins

Total Time: 9 mins

Ingredients

- 1 banana, sliced into 1/8-inch thick diagonals
- Avocado oil cooking spray

Instructions

Line air fryer basket with parchment paper.

Preheat an air fryer to 375 degrees F (190 degrees C).

Place banana slices into the basket, making sure that they are not touching; cook in batches if necessary. Mist banana slices with avocado oil.

Cook in the air fryer for 5 minutes. Remove the basket and flip banana slices carefully (they will be soft). Cook until banana slices are browning and caramelized, an additional 2 to 3 minutes. Carefully remove from basket.

Nutrition Facts

Calories:107|Protein:1.3g| Carbohydrates:27g| Fat:0.7g|
Sodium: 1.2mg.

Air Fryer Triple-Chocolate Oatmeal Cookies

Prep Time: 15 mins

Cook Time: 10 mins

Total Time: 25 mins

Ingredient

- 3 cups quick-cooking oatmeal
- 1 ½ cups all-purpose flour
- ¼ cup cocoa powder
- 1 (3.4 ounces) package instant chocolate pudding mix
- 1 teaspoon baking soda
- 1 teaspoon salt
- 1 cup butter, softened
- ¾ cup brown sugar
- ¾ cup white sugar
- 2 eggs
- 1 teaspoon vanilla extract
- 2 cups chocolate chips
- 1 cup chopped walnuts (optional)
- Nonstick cooking spray

Instructions

Preheat an air fryer to 350 degrees F (175 degrees C) according to the manufacturer's instructions. Spray the air fryer basket with nonstick cooking spray.

Mix oatmeal, flour, cocoa powder, pudding mix, baking soda, and salt in a bowl until well combined. Set aside.

Cream butter, brown sugar, and white sugar together in another bowl using an electric mixer. Add eggs and vanilla extract. Add oatmeal mixture and mix well. Stir in chocolate chips and walnuts.

Drop dough into the air fryer using a large cookie scoop; flatten out and leave about 1 inch between each cookie.

Cook until lightly browned, 6 to 10 minutes. Cool on a wire rack before serving.

Nutrition Facts

Calories: 199| Protein: 2.9g| Carbohydrates: 24.7g| Fat: 10.9g| Cholesterol: 23.9mg| Sodium: 180.4mg.

Air Fryer Beignets

Prep Time: 10 mins

Cook Time: 15 mins

Total Time: 25 mins

Ingredient

- Cooking spray
- ½ cup all-purpose flour
- ¼ cup white sugar
- ⅛ cup water
- 1 large egg, separated
- 1 ½ teaspoon melted butter
- ½ teaspoon baking powder
- ½ teaspoon vanilla extract
- 1 pinch salt
- 2 tablespoons confectioners' sugar, or to taste

Instructions

Preheat air fryer to 370 degrees F (185 degrees C). Spray a silicone egg-bite mold with nonstick cooking spray.

Whisk flour, sugar, water, egg yolk, butter, baking powder, vanilla extract, and salt together in a large bowl. Stir to combine.

Beat egg white in a small bowl using an electric hand mixer on medium speed until soft peaks form. Fold into batter. Add batter to the prepared mold using a small hinged ice cream scoop.

Place filled silicone mold into the basket of the air fryer.

Fry in the preheated air fryer for 10 minutes. Remove mold from the basket carefully; pop beignets out and flip over onto a parchment paper round.

Place parchment round with beignets back into the air fryer basket. Cook for an additional 4 minutes. Remove beignets from the air fryer basket and dust with confectioners' sugar.

Nutrition Facts

Calories: 88| Protein: 1.8g| Carbohydrates: 16.2g| Fat: 1.7g| Cholesterol: 28.9mg| Sodium: 73.5mg.

Air-Fried Banana Cake

Prep Time: 10 mins

Cook Time: 30 mins

Total Time: 40 mins

Ingredient

- Cooking spray
- ⅓ cup brown sugar
- 3 ½ tablespoons butter, at room temperature
- 1 banana, mashed
- 1 egg
- 2 tablespoons honey
- 1 cup self-rising flour
- ½ teaspoon ground cinnamon
- 1 pinch salt

Instructions

Preheat an air fryer to 320 degrees F (160 degrees C). Spray a small fluted tube pan with cooking spray.

Beat sugar and butter together in a bowl using an electric mixer until creamy. Combine banana, egg, and honey in a separate bowl. Whisk banana mixture into butter mixture until smooth.

Sift flour, cinnamon, and salt into the combined banana-butter mixture. Mix batter until smooth. Transfer to the prepared pan; level the surface using the back of a spoon.

Place the cake pan in the air fryer basket. Slide the basket into the air fryer and set the timer for 30 minutes. Bake until a toothpick inserted into the cake comes out clean.

Nutrition Facts

Calories: 497| Protein: 5.2g| Carbohydrates: 56.9g| Fat: 11.8g| Cholesterol: 73.2mg| Sodium: 530.6mg.

Air-Fried Butter Cake

Prep Time: 10 mins

Cook Time: 15 mins

Additional Time: 5 mins

Total Time: 30 mins

Ingredient

- Cooking spray
- 7 tablespoons butter, at room temperature
- ¼ cup white sugar
- 2 tablespoons white sugar
- 1 egg
- 1 ⅔ cups all-purpose flour
- 1 pinch salt, or to taste
- 6 tablespoons milk

Instructions

Preheat an air fryer to 350 degrees F (180 degrees C). Spray a small fluted tube pan with cooking spray.

Beat butter and 1/4 cup plus 2 tablespoons sugar together in a bowl using an electric mixer until light and creamy. Add egg and mix until smooth and fluffy. Stir in flour and salt. Add milk and mix batter thoroughly. Transfer batter to the prepared pan; use the back of a spoon to level the surface.

Place the pan in the air fryer basket. Set the timer for 15 minutes. Bake until a toothpick inserted into the cake comes out clean.

Turn the cake out of the pan and allow to cool for about 5 minutes.

Nutrition Facts

Calories: 470| Protein: 7.9g| Carbohydrates: 59.7g| Fat: 22.4g| Cholesterol: 101.8mg| Sodium: 209.8mg.

Don't Go Heatin' The House Gluten-Free Fresh Cherry Crumble

Prep Time: 15 mins

Cook Time: 25 mins

Additional Time: 30 mins

Total Time:1 hr 10 mins

Ingredient

- ⅓ cup butter
- 3 cups pitted cherries
- 10 tablespoons white sugar, divided
- 2 teaspoons lemon juice
- 1 cup gluten-free all-purpose baking flour
- 1 teaspoon vanilla powder
- 1 teaspoon ground nutmeg
- 1 teaspoon ground cinnamon

Instructions

Cube butter and place in freezer until firm, about 15 minutes. Preheat air fryer to 325 degrees F (165 degrees C).

Combine pitted cherries, 2 tablespoons sugar, and lemon juice in a bowl; mix well. Pour cherry mixture into baking dish.

Mix flour and 6 tablespoons of sugar in a bowl. Cut in butter using fingers until particles are pea-size. Distribute over cherries and press down lightly.

Stir 2 tablespoons sugar, vanilla powder, nutmeg, and cinnamon together in a bowl. Dust sugar topping over the cherries and flour.

Bake in the preheated air fryer. Check at 25 minutes; if not yet browned, continue cooking and checking at 5-minute intervals until slightly browned. Close drawer and turn off air fryer. Leave crumble inside for 10 minutes. Remove and allow to cool slightly, about 5 minutes.

Nutrition Facts

Calories: 459| Protein: 4.9g| Carbohydrates: 76.4g| Fat: 17.8g| Cholesterol: 40.7mg| Sodium: 109.2mg.

Easy Air Fryer Apple Pies

Prep Time: 15 mins

Cook Time: 10 mins

Total Time: 25 mins

Ingredient

- 1 (14.1 ounces) package refrigerated pie crusts (2 pie crusts)
- 1 (21 ounces) can apple pie filling
- 1 egg, beaten
- 2 tablespoons cinnamon sugar, or to taste
- 1 serving cooking spray

Instructions

Place 1 pie crust onto a lightly floured surface and roll out the dough with a rolling pin. Using a 2-1/4- inch round biscuit or cookie cutter cut the pie crust into 10 circles. Repeat with the second pie crust for a total of 20 pie crust circles.

Fill about 1/2 of each circle with apple pie filling. Place a second pie crust circle on top, making a mini pie. Do not overfill. Press down the edges of the mini pies, crimping with a fork to seal. Brush tops with beaten egg and sprinkles with cinnamon sugar.

Preheat the air fryer to 360 degrees F (175 degrees C).

Lightly spray the air fryer basket with cooking spray. Place a batch of the mini pies in the air fryer basket, leaving space around each for air circulation.

Bake until golden brown, 5 to 7 minutes. Remove from the basket and bake the remaining pies. Serve warm or at room temperature.

Nutrition Facts

Calories: 264| Protein: 2.9g| Carbohydrates: 35g| Fat: 12.8g| Cholesterol: 16.4mg| Sodium: 225mg.

Chocolate Cake In An Air Fryer

Prep Time: 10 mins

Cook Time: 15 mins

Total Time: 25 mins

Ingredient

- Cooking spray
- ¼ cup white sugar
- 3 ½ tablespoons butter, softened
- 1 egg
- 1 tablespoon apricot jam
- 6 tablespoons all-purpose flour
- 1 tablespoon unsweetened cocoa powder
- Salt to taste

Instructions

Preheat an air fryer to 320 degrees F (160 degrees C). Spray a small fluted tube pan with cooking spray.

Beat sugar and butter together in a bowl using an electric mixer until light and creamy. Add egg and jam; mix until combined.

Sift in flour, cocoa powder, and salt; mix thoroughly. Pour batter into the prepared pan. Level the surface of the batter with the back of a spoon.

Place pan in the air fryer basket. Cook until a toothpick inserted into the center of the cake comes out cleanly, about 15 minutes.

Nutrition Facts

Calories: 214| Protein: 3.2g| Carbohydrates: 25.5g| Fat: 11.7g| Cholesterol: 73.2mg| Sodium: 130.3mg.

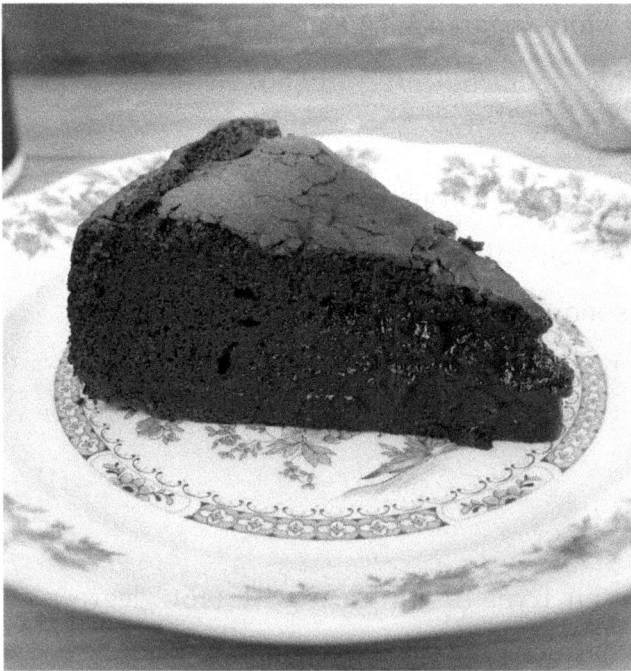

Zucchini Fries

Prep: 15 mins

Cook Time: 10 mins

Total Time: 25 mins

Ingredients

- 2 medium zucchini
- 1/2 cup flour
- 3 eggs
- Kosher salt and freshly ground black pepper
- 1/2 cup panko bread crumbs
- 1/2 cup Italian bread crumbs
- 1/4 cup parmesan cheese
- 1 Tablespoon extra virgin olive oil
- 1 teaspoon cumin Lemon Tarragon Aioli
- 1 egg
- 2 cloves garlic minced
- 3 teaspoons lemon juice plus 1 teaspoon lemon zest
- 1/2 cup canola oil
- 1/4 cup extra-virgin olive oil
- Kosher salt and freshly ground black pepper

- 2 Tablespoons minced fresh tarragon leaves

Instructions

Cut the zucchini into sticks no more than 1/2 inch thick and 3 inches long.

Add the flour to a shallow bowl. In a separate shallow bowl whisk the egg and season with salt and pepper. In a third shallow bowl, combine the panko, bread crumbs, parmesan cheese, olive oil and cumin.

Dredge zucchini in flour, then eggs, then Panko mixture. Heat air fryer to 400 degrees.

Working in batches, place the zucchini fries in a single layer in the air fryer. Cook for 8-10 minutes, until crispy. Season with kosher salt while warm.

LEMON TARRAGON AIOLI:

While the fries cooking, prepare the aioli.

Combine egg, garlic, and lemon juice in a blender or food processor. With the motor running, slowly drizzle in the canola oil until emulsified.

Transfer to a medium bowl. Whisk the aioli while slowly drizzling in the olive oil. Fold in the tarragon leaves and lemon zest and season with salt and pepper, to taste

Nutrition

Calories: 433kcal | Carbohydrates: 21g | Protein: 9g | Fat: 35g | Saturated Fat: 4g | Cholesterol: 112mg | Sodium: 285mg | Potassium: 261mg | Fiber: 1g | Sugar: 2g | Vitamin A: 340IU | Vitamin C: 13.3mg | Calcium: 108mg | Iron: 2.3mg

Air Fryer Shortbread Cookie Fries

Prep Time: 20 mins

Cook Time: 10 mins

Total Time: 30 mins

Ingredient

- 1 ¼ cups all-purpose flour
- 3 tablespoons white sugar
- ½ cup butter
- ⅓ cup strawberry jam
- ⅛ teaspoon ground dried chipotle pepper (Optional)
- ⅓ cup lemon curd

Instructions

Combine flour and sugar in a medium bowl. Cut in butter with a pastry blender until the mixture resembles fine crumbs and starts to cling. Form the mixture into a ball and knead until smooth.

Preheat an air fryer to 350 degrees F (190 degrees C).

Roll dough to 1/4-inch thickness on a lightly floured surface. Cut into 1/2-inch-wide "fries" about 3- to 4-inch long. Sprinkle with additional sugar.

Arrange fries in a single layer in the air fryer basket. Cook until lightly browned, 3 to 4 minutes. Let cool in the basket until firm enough to transfer to a wire rack to cool completely. Repeat with the remaining dough.

To make strawberry "ketchup," press jam through a fine-mesh sieve using the back of a spoon. Stir in ground chipotle. Whip the lemon curd to make it a dippable consistency for the "mustard."

Serve sugar cookie fries with strawberry ketchup and lemon curd mustard.

Nutrition Facts

Calories: 88| Protein: 0.7g| Carbohydrates: 12.4g| Fat: 4.1g| Cholesterol: 13mg| Sodium: 30.2mg.

Easy Air Fryer French Toast Sticks

Prep Time: 10 mins

Cook Time: 10 mins

Total Time: 20 mins

Ingredient

- 4 slices of slightly stale thick bread, such as Texas toast parchment paper
- 2 eggs, lightly beaten
- ¼ cup milk
- 1 teaspoon vanilla extract
- 1 teaspoon cinnamon
- 1 pinch ground nutmeg (optional)

Instructions

Cut each slice of bread into thirds to make sticks. Cut a piece of parchment paper to fit the bottom of the air fryer basket.

Preheat air fryer to 360 degrees F (180 degrees C).

Stir together eggs, milk, vanilla extract, cinnamon, and nutmeg in a bowl until well combined. Dip each piece of bread into the egg mixture, making sure each piece is well submerged. Shake each breadstick to remove excess liquid and place it in a single layer in the air fryer basket. Cook in batches, if necessary, to avoid overcrowding the fryer.

Cook for 5 minutes, turn bread pieces and cook for an additional 5 minutes.

Nutrition Facts

Calories: 232| Protein: 11.2g| Carbohydrates: 28.6g| Fat: 7.4g| Cholesterol: 188mg| Sodium: 423.4mg.

Air Fryer Peanut Butter & Jelly S'mores

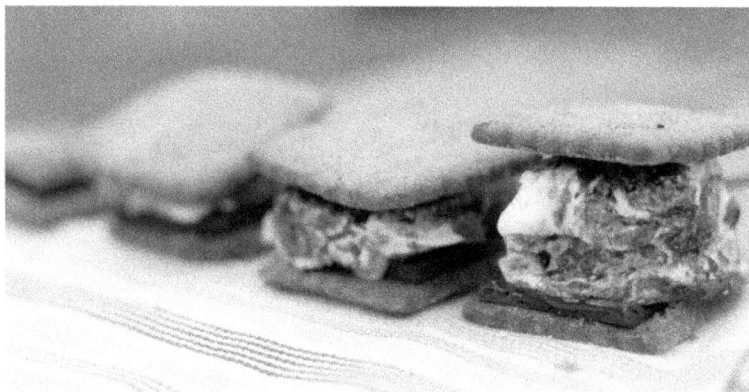

Prep Time: 5 mins

Cook Time: 5 mins

Total Time: 10 mins

Ingredient

- 1 chocolate-covered peanut butter cup
- 2 chocolate graham cracker squares, divided
- 1 teaspoon seedless raspberry jam
- 1 large marshmallow

Instructions

Preheat the air fryer to 400 degrees F (200 degrees C).

Place peanut butter cup on 1 graham cracker s◻uare. Top with jelly and marshmallow. Carefully place in an air fryer basket.

Cook in preheated air fryer until marshmallow is lightly browned and softened, about 1 minute. Immediately top with the remaining graham cracker square.

Nutrition Facts

Calories: 249| Protein: 3.9g| Carbohydrates: 41.8g| Fat: 8.2g| Cholesterol: 1mg| Sodium: 281.3mg.

Air Fryer Apple Cider Donut Bites

Prep Time: 10 mins

Cook Time: 10 mins

Additional Time: 30 mins

Total Time: 50 mins

Ingredient

- 2 ¼ cups all-purpose flour
- 3 tablespoons white sugar
- 4 teaspoons baking powder
- 1 ½ teaspoon apple pie spice
- ½ teaspoon salt
- 1 (4 ounces) container unsweetened applesauce
- ½ cup sparkling apple cider
- ¼ cup unsalted butter, melted and cooled
- 1 large egg
- 1 teaspoon apple cider vinegar

Glaze:

- teaspoon apple pie spice
- ¼ cup sparkling apple cider

- 1 teaspoon caramel extract (optional)

Instructions

Preheat the air fryer to 400 degrees F (200 degrees C) for 5 minutes.

Combine flour, sugar, baking powder, apple pie spice, and salt in a large bowl. Whisk together. Combine applesauce, sparkling apple cider, melted butter, egg, and vinegar in a small bowl; whisk until well combined. Add wet ingredients to the dry ingredients using a spatula and blend until just combined. Using a spring-hinged ice cream scoop, fill each cavity of the silicone donut mold with 2 tablespoons butter. Place the mold into the air fryer basket.

Decrease temperature to 350 degrees F (175 degrees C) and cook for 8 minutes. Carefully turn out the donut bites and cook for an additional 2 minutes.

Remove donut bites from the basket when done and let cool completely on a wire rack before glazing, about 30 minutes.

Combine powdered sugar and apple pie spice in a small bowl and whisk together. Add sparkling apple cider and caramel extract; whisk together until the glaze is smooth.

Dip each donut bite into the glaze, rolling it so that all sides are covered with the glaze. Set on a wire rack to allow the glaze to dry and harden before eating.

Nutrition Facts

Calories: 132| Protein: 1.7g| Carbohydrates: 25.9g| Fat: 2.6g| Cholesterol: 14.7mg| Sodium: 153.3mg.

Air Fryer Chocolate Chip Cookie Bites

Prep Time: 10 mins

Cook Time: 30 mins

Total Time: 40 mins

Ingredient

- ½ cup butter softened
- ½ cup packed brown sugar
- ¼ cup white sugar
- ½ teaspoon baking soda
- ½ teaspoon salt
- 1 egg
- 1 ½ teaspoons vanilla extract
- 1 ⅓ cups all-purpose flour
- 1 cup miniature semisweet chocolate chips
- ⅓ cup finely chopped pecans, toasted

Instructions

Cut a piece of parchment paper to fit an air fryer basket.

Beat butter in a large bowl with an electric mixer on medium to high speed for 30 seconds. Add brown sugar, white sugar, baking soda, and salt; beat on medium speed for 2 minutes, scraping bowl occasionally. Beat in egg and vanilla extract until combined. Add flour, beating in as much as you can. Stir in any remaining flour, chocolate chips, and pecans.

Drop dough by teaspoonfuls 1 inch apart onto the parchment paper. Carefully transfer the parchment paper to the air fryer basket.

Turn the air fryer to 300 degrees F (150 degrees C) and cook until golden brown and set about 8 minutes. Remove parchment paper to a wire rack to cool. Repeat with the remaining cookie dough.

Nutrition Facts

Calories: 188| Protein: 2g| Carbohydrates: 23.6g| Fat: 10.4g| Cholesterol: 24mg| Sodium: 150.7mg.

Easy Air Fryer Bacon and Cream Cheese Stuffed Jalapeno Poppers

Prep Time10 mins

Cook Time5 mins

Total Time15 mins

Ingredients

- 10 fresh jalapenos
- 6 oz cream cheese I used reduced-fat
- 1/4 cup shredded cheddar cheese
- 2 slices bacon cooked and crumbled
- cooking oil spray

Instructions

Slice the jalapenos in half, vertically, to create 2 halves per jalapeno. Place the cream cheese in a bowl. Microwave for 15 seconds to soften.

Remove the seeds and the inside of the jalapeno. (Save some of the seeds if you prefer spicy poppers) Combine the cream cheese, crumbled bacon, and shredded cheese in a bowl. Mix well.

For extra spicy poppers, add some of the seeds as noted above to the cream cheese mixture, and mix well.

Stuff each of the jalapenos with the cream cheese mixture.

Load the poppers into the Air Fryer. Spray the poppers with cooking oil. Close the Air Fryer. Cook the poppers on 370 degrees for 5 minutes.

Remove from the Air Fryer and cool before serving.

Air Fryer Oreos recipe!

Prep Time: 5 Minutes

Cook Time: 5 Minutes

Total Time: 10 minutes

Ingredients

8 Oreo cookies or other brand sandwich cookies

1 package Pillsbury Crescent Roll (or crescent dough sheet)

Instructions

Preheat your air fryer to 320 degrees.

Spread out crescent dough onto a cutting board or counter.

Using your finger, press down into each perforated line so it forms one big sheet. Cut the dough into eighths.

Place an Oreo cookie in the center of each of the crescent roll squares and roll each corner up (see visual above in post).

Bunch up the rest of the crescent roll to make sure it covers the entire Oreo Cookie. Do not stretch the crescent roll too thin or it will break.

Gently place the Air Fried Oreos inside the air fryer in one even row so they Do not touch. If you have a smaller air fryer, cook in batches.

Cook Oreos at 320 degrees for 5-6 minutes until golden brown on the outside.

Carefully remove the Air Fryer Oreos from the air fryer and immediately dust them with powdered sugar if desired.

Let cool for two minutes, then enjoy!

Nutrition Information

Calories: 162| Total Fat: 4g|Saturated Fat: 1g|Trans Fat: 0g|Unsaturated Fat: 1g| Cholesterol: 2mg|Sodium: 108mg|Carbohydrates: 31g|Fiber: 1g|Sugar: 21g|Protein: 2g

Air Fryer Appetizers + Easy Fried Cauliflower

Prep Time: 5 Minutes

Cook Time: 15 Minutes

Total Time: 20 Minutes

Ingredients

- 4 cups cauliflower florets
- 2 tbsp ghee, melted (or other cooking oil of choice)

Seasoning Blend:

- 2 tbsp nutritional yeast
- 1 tbsp arrowroot starch
- 1 tsp chili powder
- 1 tsp garlic powder
- 1/2 tsp smoked paprika
- 1/2 tsp sea salt

Optional Toppings:

- Chipotle aioli
- Freshly squeezed lime juice

- Fresh cilantro, chopped

Instructions

Preheat air fryer (if yours preheats) to 375° Fahrenheit and make seasoning blend. Just combine all the seasonings in a small bowl and mix. Set aside.

Chop cauliflower into florets and place in a large mixing bowl.

Add melted ghee. Toss to coat the cauliflower. Add the seasoning blend and toss again to coat.

Place cauliflower in an air fryer in an even layer with a little space between pieces. Avoid overcrowding your basket and cook in batches as needed.

Cook for 15 minutes, stirring halfway. The cauliflower will be tender and a little browned when it's done.

While cauliflower is cooking, prepare any optional toppings.

Once done, serve warm with any desired toppings, like our chipotle aioli. Enjoy.

Nutrition Value

Calories: 117kcal | Carbohydrates: 9g | Protein: 4g | Fat: 8g | Saturated Fat: 5g | Fiber: 3g

Easy Air Fryer Chicken Wings (From Frozen)

Cook Time: 30 Minutes

Total Time: 30

Ingredients

- 1.5 lbs chicken wings
- Avocado oil cooking spray
- Sea salt and pepper

For The Creamy Buffalo Sauce:

- 1 tbsp nutritional yeast
- 3 tbsp hot sauce (we like Frank's Red Hot)
- 3 tbsp mayo

Instructions

Preheat the air fryer (if yours preheats) to 400° Fahrenheit and set it to cook for 30 minutes. Note that you'll flip the wings at 10 minutes and may remove them before the 30 minutes are up. Follow the instructions below.

Place frozen chicken wings in the air fryer basket so they are in an even layer and not overlapping. Cook for 10 minutes before flipping.

While the wings are cooking, combine all of the sauce ingredients in a bowl or jar and then place in the fridge until it's time to serve.

At the end of the 10 minutes of cooking, open-air fryer, and flip wings. Cook for another 10 minutes. After a total of 20 minutes of cooking, open the air fryer again and spray wings with avocado oil cooking spray, and season with salt and pepper. Flip and spray with more avocado oil and season the other side with salt and pepper.

Continue to cook at 400° for another 5-10 minutes or until they reach your desired crispiness. Serve with creamy buffalo sauce (either on the side for dipping or toss the wings in the sauce).

Nutrition Value

Calories: 565kcal | Carbohydrates: 2g | Protein: 36g | Fat: 45g | Saturated Fat: 11g | Fiber: 1g

Air Fryer Fried Pickles (Paleo, Whole30)

Prep Time: 15 minutes

Cook Time: 10 minutes

Ingredients

- 2 cups dill pickle slices
- 1 tbsp coconut flour
- 1 large egg
- 1 cup pork panko (ground-up pork rinds)
- 1/2 tsp garlic powder
- 1/2 tsp paprika
- 1/4 tsp ground black pepper
- Sea salt, to taste see notes

Instructions

Preheat the air fryer to 400 degrees F.

Pat dry the pickle slices with a kitchen or paper towel and place in a large bowl. Sprinkle the pickles with coconut flour and toss gently so all sides are coated. In a separate bowl, crack and whisk the egg.

In another bowl, mix pork panko, garlic powder, paprika, salt, and pepper. Working in batches, dredge the pickle slices in the egg wash.

Shake off the excess and press into the pork panko mixture. Transfer to a plate and repeat with the rest of the pickle slices.

Arrange the dill pickle slices in a single layer in the air fryer. You may need to work in batches depending on the size of your air fryer.

For extra crispy pickles, spray or brush the pickles with avocado oil.

Air fry for 10 minutes, flipping then spraying (or brushing) with avocado oil again halfway through. Serve immediately with ranch, or your favorite dip!

Nutrition Facts

Fat 7g Saturated Fat 3g Cholesterol 95mg Sodium 1839mg Potassium 162mg Carbohydrates 7g Fiber 3g1

Sugar 2g Protein 13g Vitamin C 1.2mg Calcium 72mg Iron 1.2mg

Baked Sweet Potato Cauliflower Patties

Prep Time: 15

Cook Time: 20

Total Time: 35 minutes

Ingredients

- 1 medium to large sweet potato, peeled
- 2 cup cauliflower florets
- 1 green onion, chopped.
- 1 tsp minced garlic
- 2 tbsp organic ranch seasoning mix or dairy seasoning mix of choice
- 1 cup packed cilantro (fresh)
- 1/2 tsp chili powder
- 1/4 tsp cumin
- 2 tbsp arrowroot starch or gluten-free flour of choice
- 1/4 cup ground flaxseed
- 1/4 cup sunflower seeds (or pumpkin seeds)
- 1/4 tsp Kosher Salt and pepper (or to taste)
- Dipping sauce of choice

Instructions

Pre-heat oven to 400F. Line a baking sheet (or oil) and set it aside.

Next, cut your peeled sweet potato into smaller pieces. Place in a food processor or blender and pulse until the larger pieces are broken up.

Add in your cauliflower, onion, and garlic, and pulse again.

Add in your sunflower seeds, flaxseed, arrowroot (or flour), cilantro, and remaining seasonings. Pulse or place on medium until a thick batter is formed. See blog for a picture.

Place batter in a larger bowl. Scoop 1/4 cup of the batter out at a time and form into patties about 1.5 inches thick. Place on a baking sheet.

Repeat until you have about 7-10 patties.

Chill in the freeze for 10 minutes so the patties can set.

Once set, place patties in the oven for 20 minutes, flipping halfway. If you made your patties extra thick, they could take closer to 25 minutes.

Nutrition

Calories: 85 Sugar: 1.7g| Sodium: 200mg| Fat: 2.9g| Saturated Fat: 1.3g| Carbohydrates: 9g| Fiber: 3.5g| Protein: 2.7g

Keto Asparagus Fries

Prep Time: 20 mins

Cook Time: 10 mins

Resting Time: 30 mins

Total Time: 1 hr

Ingredients

- 1 pound asparagus trimmed (thick if possible)
- Salt and pepper to taste
- 1 cup Parmesan cheese
- 3/4 cup almond flour
- 1/4 teaspoon cayenne pepper
- 1/4 teaspoon baking powder
- 4 eggs beaten
- Oil spray I used avocado oil

Instructions

Using a fork, poke the asparagus spears with holes. Season well with at least 1/2 teaspoon of salt. Place on paper towels and allow to sit for 30 minutes.

Meanwhile, combine 1 cup of Parmesan, almond flour, cayenne pepper, and baking powder in a bowl. Season to taste with salt and pepper. (I use 1/4 teaspoon each.)

In a separate bowl, beat the egg.

Dip the asparagus spears in the eggs, and then coat with the cheese mixture.

Air Fryer Instructions

Preheat your air fryer to 400 degrees.

Arrange the asparagus in a single layer, cooking in batches if necessary. Spray well with oil. Cook for 5 minutes. Flip, and respray. Cook for another 4 to 5 minutes, until the asparagus, is tender.

Baked Asparagus Fries

Preheat an oven to 420 degrees. Line a baking sheet with parchment paper. Arrange the asparagus in a single layer. Spray with oil. Bake for 15 to 20 minutes.

Nutrition

Calories: 201.93kcal | Carbohydrates: 6.77g | Protein: 14.29g | Fat: 14.13g | Saturated Fat: 4.17g | Cholesterol: 120.45mg | Sodium: 310.34mg | Potassium: 225.36mg | Fiber: 3.07g | Sugar: 2.16g | Vitamin A: 894.77IU | Vitamin C: 4.23mg | Calcium: 268.52mg | Iron: 2.8mg

Keto Air Fryer Shrimp & Sweet Chili Sauce

Prep Time: 10 minutes

Cook Time: 10 minutes

Total Time: 20 minutes

Ingredients

Shrimp

- 1.5 lbs uncooked shrimp, peeled and deveined
- 1 1/3 cups almond flour
- 1/2 tsp garlic powder
- 1/2 tsp onion powder
- 1 tsp paprika
- 1/2 tsp sea salt
- 1/4 tsp pepper 2 tsp parsley
- 1 large egg, beaten

Chili Sauce

- 1 1/2 tsp red pepper flakes
- 1/2 cup apple cider vinegar
- 1/2 cup water

- 1 1/2 tbsp coconut aminos
- 1/2 cup powdered sweetener (Swerve or Monk Fruit)
- 1 tsp ground ginger
- 1/4 tsp salt
- 2 tsp minced garlic
- 1/4 tsp xanthan gum

Instructions

Air Fryer Shrimp

Preheat the air fryer to 380 degrees.

In a medium bowl, add the almond flour, garlic powder, onion powder, paprika, parsley, and salt/ pepper and mix.

In a small bowl, add the beaten egg.

Dip each shrimp in the egg then the flour mixture. Place on a plate until all shrimp are completely coated.

Spray the air fryer basket with cooking spray and add the shrimp to where they are not touching (You may have to cook in 2 batches).

Spray the top of the shrimp with cooking spray and set the air fryer to 380F and cook for 9-10 minutes making sure to flip the shrimp halfway through. Once flipped, spray the shrimp with another round of cooking spray.

Sweet Chili Sauce

In a small saucepan, add all of the sauce ingredients except the xanthan gum. Heat over medium/high heat and bring to a boil.

Reduce heat to low and add in the xanthan gum and stir until combined. Add to a jar and store in the fridge for up to 2 weeks.

Nutrition

Calories: 290| Sugar: 1g| Sodium: 395mg| Fat: 6g| Carbohydrates: 6| Fiber: 2| Protein: 31g| Cholesterol: 219mg

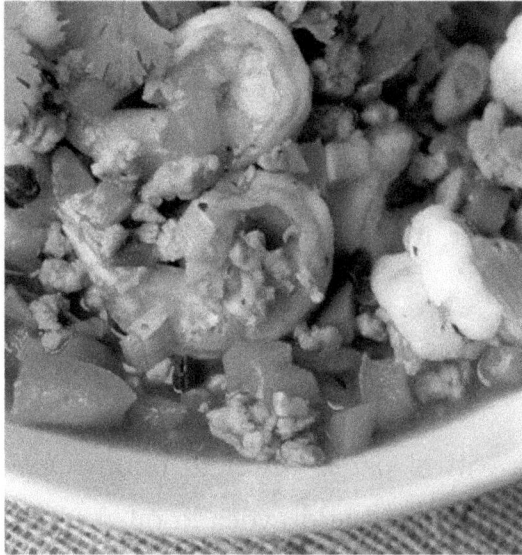

Air Fryer Buffalo Wings

Prep Time: 5 minutes

Cook Time: 45 minutes

Total Time: 50 minutes

Ingredients

- 1 1/2 pounds chicken wings (about 16 wings)
- 1 tablespoon avocado oil
- 1 1/2 teaspoons garlic powder
- 1 1/2 teaspoons paprika
- 1/2-3/4 teaspoon cayenne pepper
- 1/3 cup homemade buffalo sauce (or more for your liking)
- Salt and pepper, to taste

Instructions

Pat dry wings with a paper towel to remove excess moisture. Add to a large bowl and add avocado oil, 1 tablespoon buffalo sauce, garlic powder, paprika, cayenne, and salt and pepper. Mix well to combine. If desired, spray the bottom of your air fryer basket with oil (I used avocado oil spray). Place wings in your air fryer basket, evenly spreading out and leaving a little room in between them so the air can easily flow through. Close drawer set air fryer on manual at 400°F for 22 minutes. Depending on the size of your air fryer, you will probably have to cook the wings in two batches to make sure they are not overcrowded.

When the wings are almost done, either make or heat the buffalo sauce.

Once wings are done, add to a large bowl and pour buffalo sauce over wings. Carefully mix to coat the wings. Serve with ranch or blue cheese, carrots, celery, and more hot sauce, and enjoy immediately

Nutrition Facts

Fat: 27g Saturated: Fat 9g

Polyunsaturated Fat: 1g

Monounsaturated Fat: 3g Potassium: 8mg

Protein: 30g Vitamin C: 1mg Calcium: 3mg

Air Fryer Potato Wedges

Prep Time: 5 Minutes

Cook Time: 15 Minutes

Soaking Time: 30 Minutes

Total Time: 50 Minutes

Ingredients

- 2 medium Russet potatoes, cut into wedges
- 1 1/2 Tbsp olive oil
- 1/2 tsp paprika
- 1/4 tsp garlic powder
- 1/8 tsp cayenne pepper, (optional)
- 1 tsp sea salt
- 1/4 tsp ground black pepper

Instructions

Place raw potato wedges in a bowl and add cold water and 2 cups of ice cubes. Let them soak for at least 30 min then drain them and pat them dry with paper towels.

Preheat Air Fryer if it is recommended for your model.

In a large bowl or ziplock bag combine olive oil, paprika, garlic powder, cayenne pepper, salt, and black pepper. Add the potato wedges and toss to coat the potatoes with the seasoning.

Place wedges in the basket of the air fryer and cook for 15 minutes at 400F (200C). Shaking the basket every 5 minutes. Depending on your Air Fryer you might have to fry them in batches.

In a bowl combine grated Parmesan cheese and parsley if using. Transfer cooked wedges to the bowl and toss until coated with the topping. Serve with ketchup or sour cream on the side.

Nutrition Information

Calories: 187kcal | Carbohydrates: 20g | Protein: 7g | Fat: 9g | Saturated Fat: 3g | Cholesterol: 11mg | Sodium: 779mg | Potassium: 460mg | Fiber: 1g | Sugar: 1g | Vitamin A: 330iu | Vitamin C: 7mg | Calcium: 152mg | Iron: 1mg

Crispy Air Fryer Cauliflower

Prep Time: 2 Minutes

Cook Time: 13 Minutes

Total Time: 15 Minutes

Ingredients

- 1 bag Trader Joe's Cauliflower Gnocchi
- Cooking oil spray

Instructions

Spread the frozen Trader Joe's Cauliflower gnocchi on a microwave-safe plate. Microwave for 1 minute (if using the whole bag). Flip halfway to make sure they are thawed evenly.

Toss the cauliflower gnocchi in the air fryer basket. Lightly spray with cooking oil. Cook 400 F for 13 - 15 minutes.

Pair with your favorite sauce or sides. Enjoy!

Nutrition Information

Calories: 97|Total Fat: 1g|Saturated Fat: 0g|Trans Fat: 0g|Unsaturated Fat: 1g|Cholesterol: 9mg|Sodium: 26mg|Carbohydrates: 19g| Fiber: 4g|Sugar: 3g|Protein: 5g

Air Fryer Green Bean Fries

Prep Time: 5 minutes

Cook Time: 9 minutes

Total Time: 14 minutes

Ingredients

- 1 pound of green beans, ends trimmed
- 1 large egg
- 3/4 cup almond flour
- 2 tablespoons nutritional yeast
- 1 teaspoon garlic powder
- 1 teaspoon onion powder
- 3/4 tsp salt

Instructions

Preheat air fryer to 390°F. Trim the ends of the green beans and rinse/dry.

Prepare your two dipping bowls. One for the egg wash and the other with all the dry ingredients One at a time, dip green beans in the egg wash and then the dry mix.

Place in an air fryer in an even layer and spray the beans with cooking spray. Cook for 8-9 minutes until golden brown. At the halfway mark, be sure to shake the basket and spray the tops with cooking spray to help get a crunch texture,

Serve with my homemade ranch dressing.

Nutrition

Calories: 148 Sugar: 3g| Sodium: 371mg| Fat: 4g| Carbohydrates: 10g| Fiber: 3g| Protein: 6g| Cholesterol: 37mg

Air Fryer Bang Bang Chicken

Prep Time: 10 Minutes

Cook Time: 20 Minutes

Ingredients

Bang Bang Chicken

- 1 lb chicken breast (cut into 1-inch pieces)
- 1 cup blanched almond flour
- 1/2 cup crushed plantain chips or tortilla chips
- 1/2 tsp sea salt
- 1 large egg
- 1 tbsp lime juice

Bang Bang Sauce

- 1/2 cup mayonnaise
- 1 tbsp chili garlic sauce
- 1 tbsp rice vinegar
- 1 tbsp honey

Instructions

Begin by prepping the chicken. In a shallow bowl, combine the almond flour, salt, and crushed up chips.

In a separate bowl, whisk together lime juice and egg.

Take each chicken piece and dip it into the egg mixture first, then dip it into the flour/chip mixture. Place all chicken pieces in one layer in the air fryer (you may have to do it in batches if you have a small air fryer).

Set the air fryer to 380 and cook for 8-10 minutes, or until chicken is cooked through. Flip over each chicken piece, and cook for another 6-8 minutes, or until nice and crispy.

While chicken is cooking, make the sauce. In a small bowl, whisk together the mayonnaise, chili garlic sauce, honey, and rice vinegar.

Once the chicken is done place it on a large plate and drizzle with sauce. You can also use it as a dipping sauce.

For The Oven:

Preheat the oven to 450 degrees while you prepare the chicken. Lightly grease a large sheet pan. Place each chicken piece on the sheet pan and bake for 12 minutes, flip over the chicken, and bake another 10-12 minutes.

Nutritional Value

Calories: 589kcal| Fat: 42g| Saturated Fat: 6g| Cholesterol: 131mg| Sodium: 887mg| Potassium: 468mg| Carbohydrates: 21g| Fiber: 4g| Sugar: 7g| Protein: 33g

Air Fryer Zucchini

Prep Time: 5 Minutes

Cook Time: 20 Minutes

Total Time: 25 Minutes

Ingredients

- 2 medium zucchinis
- 1/2 cup shredded Parmesan
- 1 egg
- 2 heaping tbsp avocado oil
- 1/2 cup almond flour
- 2 tbsp coconut flour
- 1/2 tsp garlic powder
- 1/4 tsp smoked paprika
- Salt pepper to taste

Instructions

Wash and dry zucchinis. Cut into strips about 3 inches long.A bowl of zucchinis cut into strips.

In a shallow bowl, whisk together egg and avocado oil. In a separate bowl, whisk together almond flour, coconut flour, parmesan, and seasoning. Instruction on how to make air fryer zucchini fries, step by step.

Dredge zucchini slices in the egg mixture. Then evenly coat zucchini slices with flour mixture. Make sure all surfaces are coated.

Next, spray the air fryer basket then place zucchini slices in it with a little bit of space in between. Basket of zucchini fries before frying in the air fryer. Make sure to not overcrowd them. If they are too close or overlapping they won't cook properly. (I used a rack so you can cook more in one batch)

Fry in the air fryer at 400 F for 9-10 minutes

Nutrition Information

Calories: 220| Total Fat: 18g| Saturated Fat: 3g| Trans Fat: 0g| Unsaturated Fat: 14g| Cholesterol: 50mg| Sodium: 254mg| Carbohydrates: 9g| Fiber: 3g| Sugar: 3g| Protein: 9g

Air Fryer Chicken Kiev Balls

Prep Time: 15 mins

Cook Time: 10 mins

Additional Time: 30 mins

Total Time: 55 mins

Ingredient

- ½ Cup unsalted butter softened
- 2 tablespoons chopped fresh flat-leaf parsley
- 2 cloves garlic, crushed
- 1 (19.1 ounces) package ground chicken breast
- 2 eggs, beaten
- 1 cup panko bread crumbs 1 teaspoon paprika
- 1 teaspoon salt
- ½ teaspoon ground black pepper
- Cooking spray

Instructions

Mix butter, parsley, and garlic in a bowl until evenly combined.

Divide mixture into 12 equal parts on a baking sheet. Freeze until solid, about 20 minutes.

Shape ground chicken into 12 balls. Make a deep thumbprint in the center of each ball. Place a piece of frozen herbed butter in the indention and wrap the meat around the butter until it is fully encased. Repeat with the remaining balls.

Place beaten eggs in a bowl. Combine panko, paprika, salt, and pepper in a separate bowl.

Dip 1 ground chicken ball first in the beaten eggs, then in the seasoned bread crumbs. Dip the ball back into the egg and in the seasoned bread crumbs once more. Repeat with the remaining balls. Place on a baking sheet and freeze for 10 minutes.

Preheat an air fryer to 400 degrees F (200 degrees C). Place 1/2 of the balls in the air fryer basket and spray with nonstick cooking spray.

Cook for 5 minutes. Flip balls over with tongs and spray again with nonstick cooking spray. Cook for 5 minutes more. Repeat with remaining chicken balls.

Nutrition Facts

Calories:154|Protein:12.6g| Carbohydrates: 6.7g| Fat: 9.4g| Cholesterol: 77.5mg| Sodium: 280.3mg

Air Fryer Roasted Salsa

Prep Time: 15 mins

Cook Time: 10 mins

Additional Time:10 mins

Total Time: 35 mins

Ingredient

- 4 Roma tomatoes, halved lengthwise
- 1 jalapeno pepper, halved and seeded
- ½ red onion, cut into 2 wedges
- Cooking spray
- 4 cloves garlic, peeled
- ½ cup chopped cilantro
- 1 lime, juiced
- Salt to taste

Instructions

Preheat the air fryer to 390 degrees F (200 degrees C).

Place tomatoes and jalapeno skin-side down into the air fryer basket, along with the red onion. Lightly spray vegetables with cooking spray to help the roasting process.

Air fry vegetables for 5 minutes. Open the basket and add garlic cloves. Spray lightly with cooking spray and air fry for an additional 5 minutes.

Transfer vegetables to a cutting board and allow to cool for 10 minutes.

Remove skins from tomatoes and jalapeno, if desired; they should slip right off. Chop tomatoes, jalapeno, and onion into large chunks and add to the bowl of a food processor. Add garlic, cilantro, lime juice, and salt. Pulse several times until vegetables are finely chopped; do not over-process. Serve at room temperature or refrigerate to let flavors meld.

Nutrition Facts

Calories: 30;   Protein: 1.3g|Carbohydrates:6.8g| Fat:0.3g|Sodium:33.5mg

Air Fryer Green Beans

Prep Time: 5 mins

Cook Time: 10 mins

Total Time: 15 mins

Ingredients

- 1 lb green beans
- 1 tbsp olive oil
- 1/2 tsp salt
- 1/4 tsp pepper

Instructions

Trim the green beans, then toss with olive oil, salt, and pepper.

Put prepared green beans in the air fryer basket and cook at 400F for 10 minutes, shaking the basket halfway through.

Nutrition

Calories: 66kcal | Carbohydrates: 8g | Protein: 2g | Fat: 4g | Saturated Fat: 1g | Sodium: 298mg | Potassium: 239mg | Fiber: 3g | Sugar: 4g | Vitamin A: 782IU | Vitamin C: 14mg | Calcium: 42mg | Iron: 1mg

Healthy Air Fryer Chicken and Veggies (20 Minutes!)

Prep Time: 5 minutes

Cook Time: 15 minutes

Total Time: 20 minutes

Ingredients

- 1 pound chicken breast, chopped into bite-size pieces (2-3 medium chicken breasts)
- 1 cup broccoli florets (fresh or frozen)
- 1 zucchini chopped
- 1 cup bell pepper chopped (any colors you like)
- 1/2 onion chopped
- 2 cloves garlic minced or crushed
- 2 tablespoons olive oil
- 1/2 teaspoon EACH garlic powder, chili powder, salt, pepper
- 1 tablespoon Italian seasoning (or spice blend of choice)

Instructions

Preheat air fryer to 400F.

Chop the veggies and chicken into small bite-size pieces and transfer to a large mixing bowl. Add the oil and seasoning to the bowl and toss to combine.

Add the chicken and veggies to the preheated air fryer and cook for 10 minutes, shaking halfway, or until the chicken and veggies are charred and chicken is cooked through. If your air fryer is small, you may have to cook them in 2-3 batches.

Nutrition

Serving: 1serving | Calories: 230kcal | Carbohydrates: 8g | Protein: 26g | Fat: 10g | Saturated Fat: 2g | Cholesterol: 73mg | Sodium: 437mg | Potassium: 734mg | Fiber: 3g | Sugar: 4g | Vitamin A: 1584IU | Vitamin C: 79mg | Calcium: 50mg | Iron: 1mg

Fried Green Beans (Air Fryer)

Prep Time: 5 minutes

Cook Time: 5 minutes

Total Time: 10 minutes

Ingredients

- 1 lb. fresh green beans (cleaned and trimmed)
- 1 tsp. oil
- 1/4 tsp. garlic powder
- 1/8 tsp. sea salt

Instructions

Toss all the ingredients together in a bowl to coat the green beans with oil and spices.

Transfer about half of the green beans to the air fryer basket. (You'll have to do this in two batches or the beans won't cook properly) Spread them out as evenly as possible and return the basket to the air fryer.

Adjust temp to 400 and set time to 5 minutes, or whichever time you chose from the chart above, and press start.

When done, remove the basket from the fryer and turn the beans out onto a platter (repeat with the second half of the beans).

If you try the beans and they aren't cooked enough to your liking, simply return them to the air fryer in the basket and cook in 2-minute increments until they are cooked to your liking.

Cool slightly and serve.

Nutrition

Serving: 0.25the recipe | Calories: 47kcal | Carbohydrates: 8g | Protein: 2g | Fat: 1g | Saturated Fat: 1g | Sodium: 67mg | Potassium: 239mg | Fiber: 3g | Sugar: 4g | Vitamin A: 782IU | Vitamin C: 14mg | Calcium: 42mg | Iron: 1mg

Air Fryer Green Beans

Prep Time: 5 mins

Cook Time: 15 mins

Total Time: 20 mins

Ingredients

- 1 pound (454 g) fresh green beans, ends trimmed and halved
- 1-2 tablespoons (15 ml) olive oil or spray
- 1/2 teaspoon (2.5 ml) garlic powder
- Salt and pepper, to taste
- Fresh lemon slices

Instructions

In a bowl, combine green beans, oil, garlic powder, salt, and pepper. Place the seasoned green beans in an air fryer basket.

Air Fry 360°F for about 10-14 minutes depending on your preferred doneness. Toss and shake about 2 times during cooking.

Season with salt and pepper, to taste. Serve with lemon slices or wedges

Nutrition

Calories: 67kcal | Carbohydrates: 8g | Protein: 2g | Fat: 4g |
Saturated Fat: 1g | Sodium: 7mg | Potassium: 239mg | Fiber: 3g
| Sugar: 4g | Vitamin A: 782IU | Vitamin C: 14mg | Calcium:
42mg | Iron: 1mg

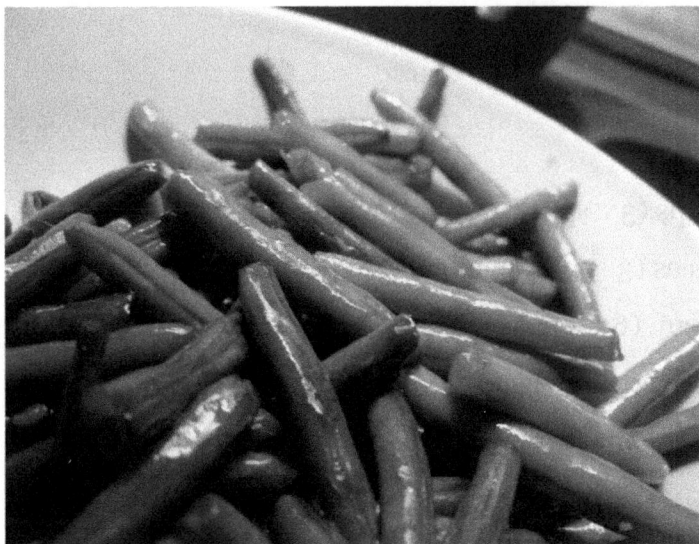

Air Fryer Green Beans With Bacon

Prep Time: 15 minutes

Cook Time: 10 minutes

Total Time: 25 minutes

Ingredients

- 3 cups (330 g) Frozen Cut Green Beans
- 3 slices (3 slices) bacon, diced
- 1/4 cup (62.5 ml) Water
- 1 teaspoon (1 teaspoon) Kosher Salt
- 1 teaspoon (1 teaspoon) Ground Black Pepper

Instructions

Place the frozen green beans, onion, bacon, and water in a 6 x 3-inch heatproof pan. Place the pan in the air fryer basket. Set air fryer to 375°F for 15 minutes.

Raise the air fryer temperature to 400°F for 5 minutes. Add salt and pepper to taste and toss well. Remove from the air fryer and cover the pan. Let it rest for 5 minutes and serve.

I find that frozen vegetables often cook up better in an air fryer if you're looking for moist, tender beans.

If you want crispy beans, you should start with fresh beans rather than frozen. You can also substitute cooked sausage for the bacon.

If you use lean chicken sausage, then you may have to spray the beans with a little oil to get the best "air-fried" texture from them.

Nutrition

Calories: 95kcal | Carbohydrates: 6g | Protein: 3g | Fat: 6g | Fiber: 2g | Sugar: 2g

Air Fryer Stuffed Peppers

Prep Time: 15 Minutes

Cook Time: 15 Minutes

Total Time: 30 Minutes

Ingredients

- 6 Green Bell Peppers
- 1 Lb Lean Ground Beef
- 1 Tbsp Olive Oil
- 1/4 Cup Green Onion Diced
- 1/4 Cup Fresh Parsley
- 1/2 Tsp Ground Sage
- 1/2 Tsp Garlic Salt
- 1 Cup Cooked Rice
- 1 Cup Marinara Sauce More to Taste
- 1/4 Cup Shredded Mozzarella Cheese

Instructions

Warm-up a medium-sized skillet with the ground beef and cook until well done. Drain the beef and return to the pan.

Add in the olive oil, green onion, parsley, sage, and salt. Mix this well. Add in the cooked rice and marinara, mix well.

Cut the top off of each pepper and clean the seeds out.

Scoop the mixture into each of the peppers and place it in the basket of the air fryer. (I did 4 the first round, 2 the second to make them fit.)

Cook for 10 minutes at 355*, carefully open and add cheese.

Cook for an additional 5 minutes or until peppers are slightly soft and cheese is melted. Serve.

Nutrition Information

Calories: 296| Total Fat: 13g| Saturated Fat: 4g| Trans Fat: 0g| Unsaturated Fat: 7g| Cholesterol: 70mg| Sodium: 419mg| Carbohydrates: 19g| Fiber: 2g| Sugar: 6g| Protein: 25g

Air Fryer Weight Watchers Stuffed Peppers

Prep Time: 5 Mins

Cook Time: 25 Mins

Total Time: 30 Mins

Ingredients

- 6 bell peppers red, yellow, and orange
- 1/4 cup water
- 1/2 lb ground turkey breast LEAN
- 1 small zucchini small dice
- 2 cups crushed tomatoes no salt added
- 1 cup mushrooms small dice
- 1.5 cups cauliflower rice
- 1 tbsp Worcestershire sauce
- 1 tsp salt
- 3 Babybel Mini Light Cheese Rounds grated

Instructions

Heat non-stick skillet on medium-high

Add water, ground turkey, zucchini, and mushrooms Brown for five minutes and add salt

While turkey is browning, heat cauliflower rice in microwave according to package directions To the turkey, add Worcestershire, rice, and tomatoes and simmer for 2-3 minutes

While turkey mixture is cooking, prep peppers by slicing off tops and clean the insides (save the pepper tops to use in other recipes)

Spoon turkey mixture into peppers

Air Fryer Instructions: AF at 350 for 10 minutes. Open AF and add shredded cheese. Air Fry 5 minutes more until cheese melts and browns

Oven Instructions: Cover with foil and bake at 350 for 30 minutes. Uncover and add shredded cheese. Bake an additional 15 minutes (uncovered)

Nutrition Value

Calories: 400kcal Carbohydrates: 27g Protein: 66.1g

Fat: 4.4g Saturated Fat: 1.3g Cholesterol: 146mg Sodium: 1118mg Potassium: 520mg Fiber: 7.4g

Sugar: 18g Calcium: 211mg Iron: 3mg

Easy Air Fryer Parmesan-Crusted Tilapia

Prep Time: 3 Mins

Cook Time: 7 Mins

Total Time: 10 Mins

Ingredients

- 2 thin tilapia fillets (about 4 ounces) fresh or frozen (times given for both below)
- Olive oil pump spray not aerosol or 1 tablespoon olive oil
- 1/4 teaspoon salt
- 1/4 teaspoon ground pepper (optional)
- 2 tablespoons grated Parmesan cheese
- 1/2 cup fine dry breadcrumbs

Instructions

Place the frozen tilapia fillets on an aluminum or stainless steel baking pan while preheating the air fryer and measuring ingredients.

Crazy Good Tip: These few minutes on the baking pan will ever so slightly thaw the fillets just enough to allow the breadcrumbs to stick to the oil on them. Preheat the air fryer to 390-400 degrees for 3 minutes. Most air fryers preset "air fryer" button is 390F to 400F degrees.

Spray or coat fish fillets with olive oil sprayer or mister or brush with olive oil. (Not Pam aerosol vegetable cooking spray)

Sprinkle both sides of fillets with salt and if desired, pepper. Sprinkle the top side of fillets with Parmesan cheese.

Place the dry breadcrumbs on a plate and gently press the fish into the breadcrumbs to coat them. If you have trouble getting the breadcrumbs to stick to the fish, wait just a few minutes or I like to spray the breaded fish again on top with a little bit of olive oil spray (again, not aerosol) Frozen fish: Air Fry at 390-400 degrees for 9 to 11 minutes, without turning, depending on the thickness of fish until fish flakes easily in the center.

Fresh fish: Air Fry at 390-400 degrees for 7 minutes, without turning, depending on the thickness of fish until fish flakes easily in the center.

Carefully remove the fish with a silicone-coated spatula to prevent scraping the nonstick surface.

Nutrition Value

Calories: 206kcal

Air Fryer Steak Bites & Mushrooms

Prep Time: 10 mins

Cook Time: 18 mins

Total Time: 28 mins

Ingredients

- 1 lb. (454 g) steaks, cut into 1/2" cubes (ribeye, sirloin, tri-tip, or what you prefer)
- 8 oz. (227 g) mushrooms (cleaned, washed, and halved)
- 2 tablespoons (30 ml) butter, melted (or olive oil)
- 1 teaspoon (5 ml) worcestershire sauce
- 1/2 teaspoon (2.5 ml) garlic powder, optional
- Flakey salt, to taste
- Fresh cracked black pepper, to taste
- Minced parsley, garnish
- Melted butter, for finishing - optional
- Chili flakes, for finishing - optional

Instructions

Rinse and thoroughly pat dry the steak cubes. Combine the steak cubes and mushrooms. Coat with the melted butter and then season with Worcestershire sauce, optional garlic powder, and a generous seasoning of salt and pepper.

Preheat the Air Fryer at 400°F for 4 minutes.

Spread the steak and mushrooms in an even layer in the air fryer basket. Air fry at 400°F for 10-18 minutes, shaking and flipping and the steak and mushrooms 2 times through the cooking process (time depends on your preferred doneness, the thickness of the steak, size of air fryer).

Check the steak to see how well done it is cooked. If you want the steak more done, add an extra 2-5 minutes of cooking time.

Garnish with parsley and drizzle with optional melted butter and/or optional chili flakes. Season with additional salt & pepper if desired. Serve warm.

Nutrition Value

Calories: 401kcal | Carbohydrates: 3g | Protein: 32g | Fat: 29g | Saturated Fat: 14g | Cholesterol: 112mg| Sodium: 168mg | Potassium: 661mg | Sugar: 1g | Vitamin C: 1.6mg | Calcium: 11mg | Iron: 3.1mg

Air Fryer Plantain Chips

Prep Time: 5 Mins

Cook Time: 12 Mins

Total Time: 17 Mins

Ingredients

- 1 Green Plantain Evenly sliced
- 1 Tsp. Kosher Salt or to taste
- 1 Cup Water
- Lemon or Lime Juice Optional

Instructions

Add the water and salt to a bowl. Stir. Set aside. Peel the plantains.

Sliced the plantains in even slices. Best to use a mandolin.

Add the plantain slices to the salted water, let soak for about 5-10 minutes.

Transfer to the air fryer. Spray with olive oil, cook for 12 minutes, shaking and spraying with oil in between cooking.

Increase the time for desired crispiness. Sprinkle with lemon or lime juice (optional). Enjoy!

Nutrition Value

Calories: 537kcal Carbohydrates: 141g Protein: 3g

Fat: 2g

Sodium: 1147mg Potassium: 2163mg Fiber: 8g

Sugar: 78g Vitamin A: 120IU Vitamin C: 165mg Calcium: 10mg Iron: 18mg

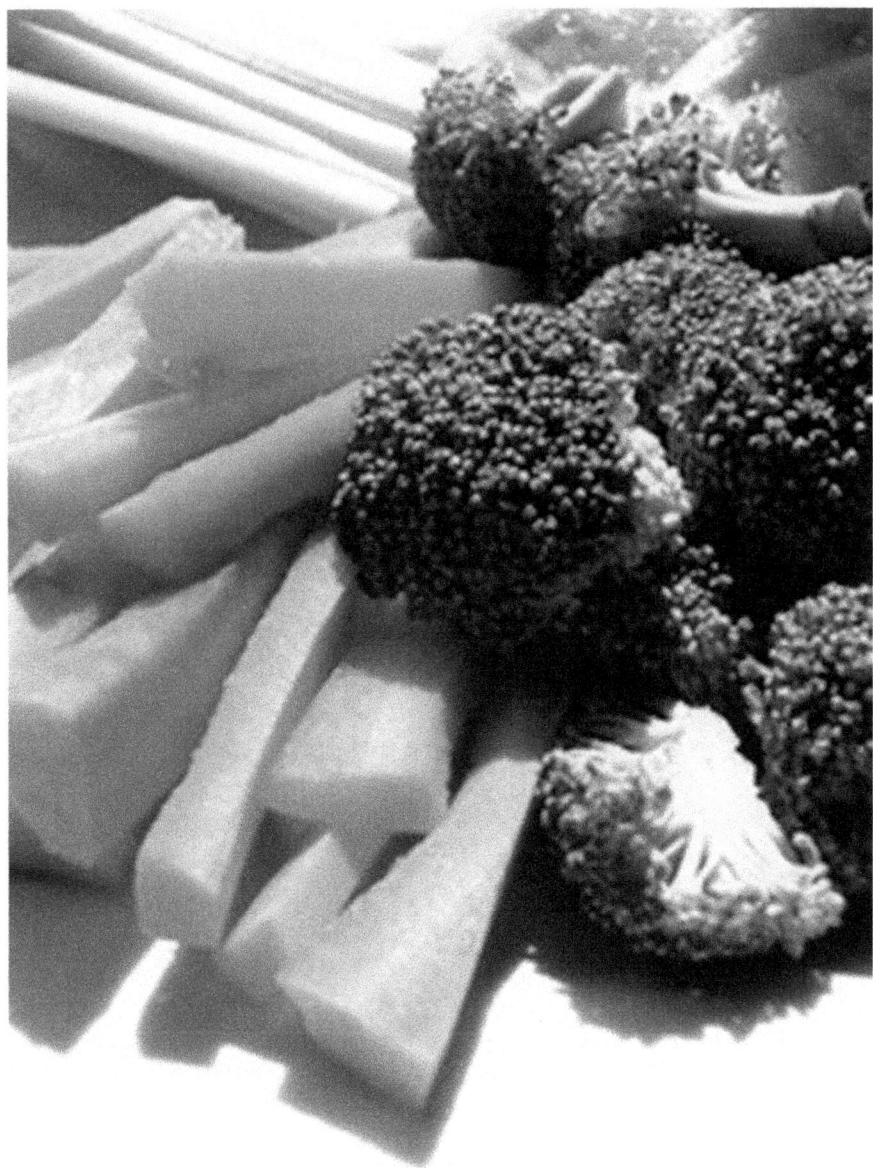

www.ingramcontent.com/pod-product-compliance
Lightning Source LLC
Chambersburg PA
CBHW050748030426
42336CB00012B/1719